The 8 Laws of Health
A Coloring and Activity Book for Children

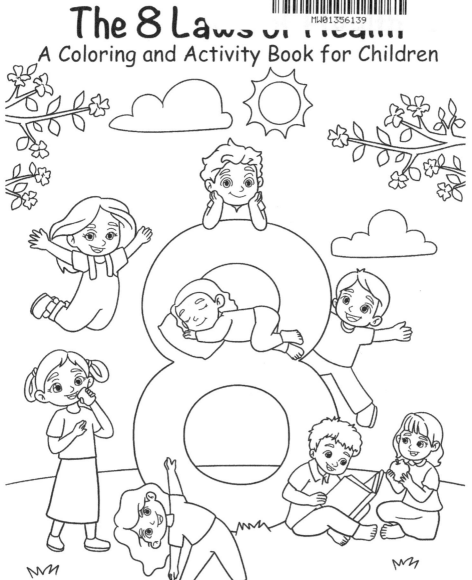

This Amazing Health Treasure Belongs to:

_____

Copyright
Copyright © 2024 by PureBlue Publications
Printed in the United States of America
All rights reserved.

Scripture quotations are taken from the
Holy Bible, King James Version

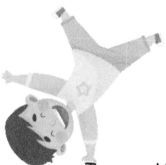

Terase Wallace, RN

Cover designed by Rocel Hernandez
Interior Illustration by Rocel Hernandez
Reviewed by Sadae Evans

EarnestInk Publications

www.earnestink.com
earnestinkpress@gmail.com

Come along on this exciting journey through the 8 Laws of Health!

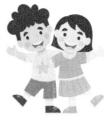

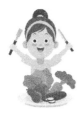

Nutrition!

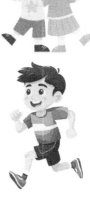

Exercise!

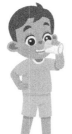

Water!

Sunlight!

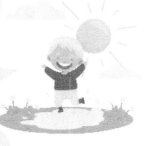

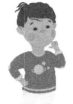

Temperance!

Air!

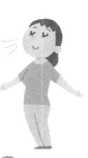

Rest!

Trust in GOD!

The 8 Laws of Health use the acronym:

N – Nutrition
E – Exercise
W – Water
S – Sunlight
T – Temperance
A – Air
R – Rest
T – Trust in God

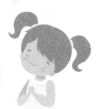

"I can do all things through Christ who strengthens me."
Philippians 4:13

N E W S T A R T

NEWSTART is a registered trademark
of Weimar University, used by permission

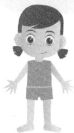
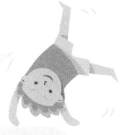

Our beautiful bodies were created by God.

Can you name the parts of your body?

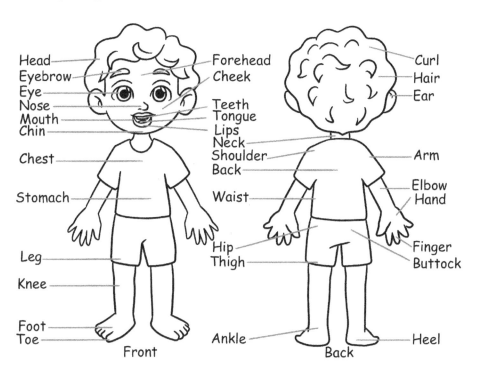

"I will praise thee; for I am fearfully and wonderfully made; marvelous are your works; and that my soul knows right well."
Psalm 139:14

NUTRITION

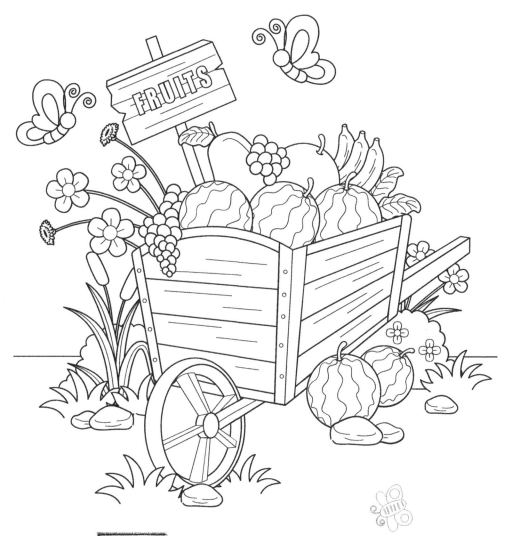

"Whether therefore ye eat, or drink, or whatsoever ye do, do all to the glory of God."
I Corinthians 10:31

Why is it important for us to eat fruits and vegetables?

They have vitamin C, which strengthens our bones and teeth and helps us run, jump, and play!

Eating different kinds of colorful fruits and vegetables protects us from diseases.

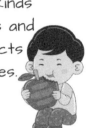

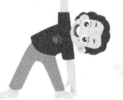

Fruits give us the energy we need to play, learn, and explore.

They have many nutrients that help our bodies grow healthy and strong.

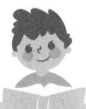

They help our brains work better to become smarter.

What is your favorite fruit?

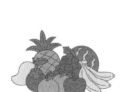

_____

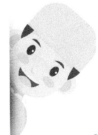

Eating lots of fruits, veggies, nuts, beans, and seeds keeps us healthy and strong!

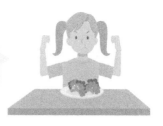

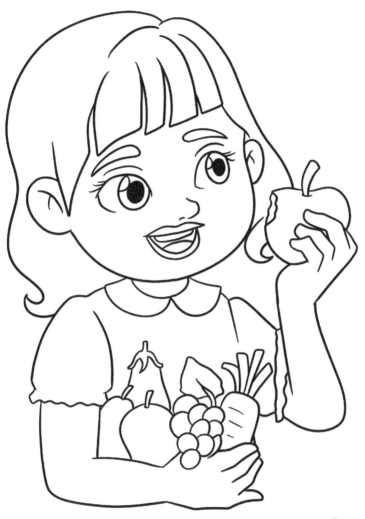

Eat healthy; be happy!

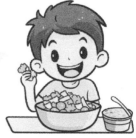

Fun Facts:

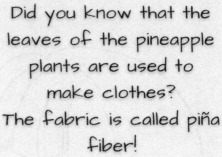

Did you know that the leaves of the pineapple plants are used to make clothes? The fabric is called piña fiber!

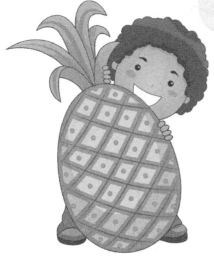

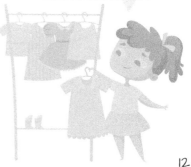

Wow! That's so cool!

The food we eat can change how our body and brain feel!

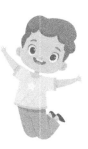

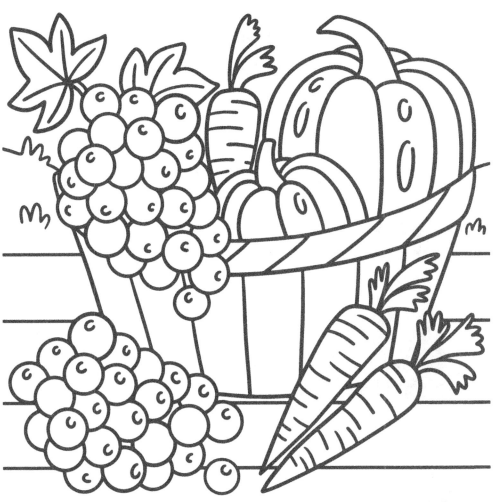

Eating fruits, veggies, nuts, beans, and seeds helps us solve problems quickly and correctly!

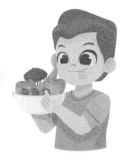

Fun Facts:

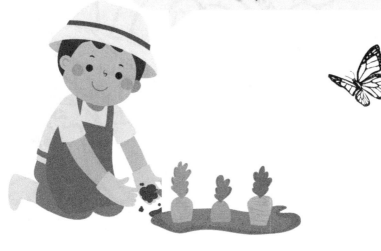

Did you know that carrots are made up of 88% water?

Yes, they are!
They also come in different colors, like orange, purple, red, white, yellow, and black.
Enjoy them all!

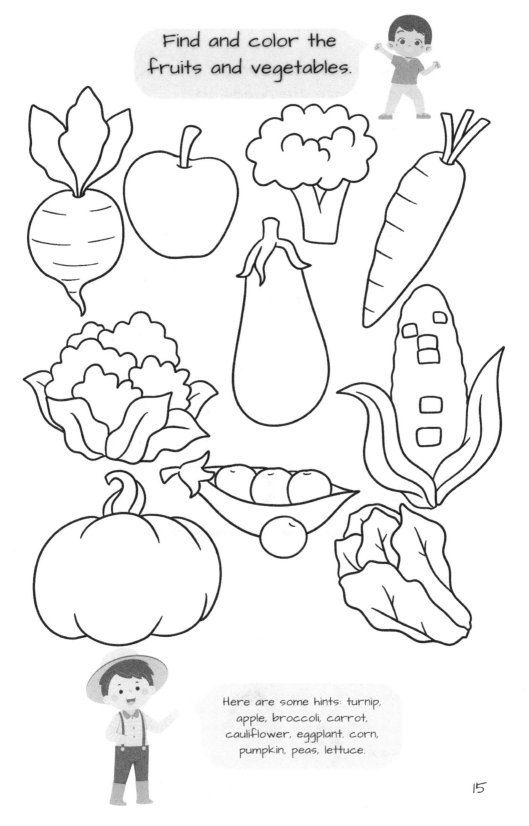

Help Carson find his way through the maze. He needs to get the apple to take to school!

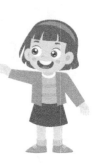

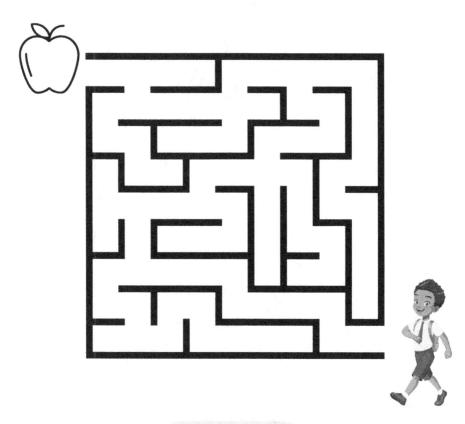

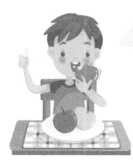

An apple a day keeps the doctor away!

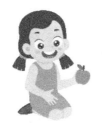

It is very important to choose healthy foods to eat!

Healthy Food   Unhealthy Food

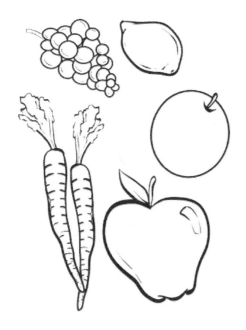
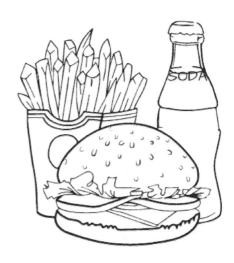

What are the right choices I should make?

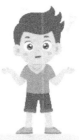

I choose healthy foods for me, to stay as healthy as can be.

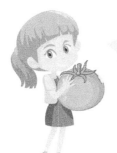

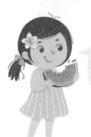

The healthiest foods are those that come from a plant.

Draw lines to connect all the healthy foods to the center circle.

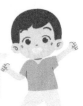

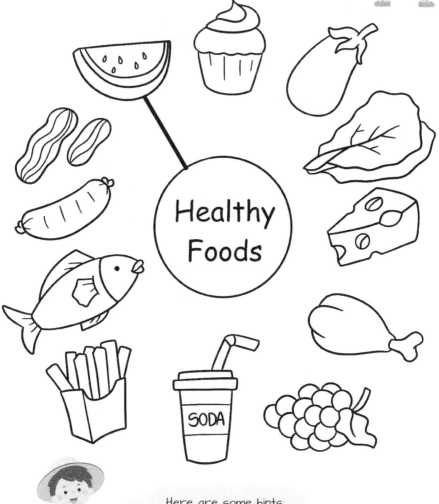

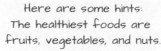

Here are some hints: The healthiest foods are fruits, vegetables, and nuts.

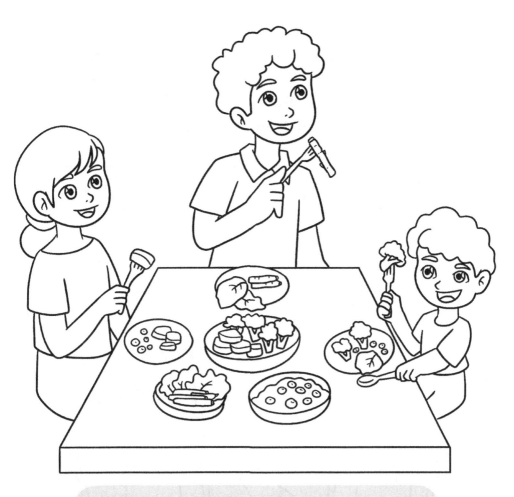

Make sure most of your meal is filled with fruits or veggies, like carrots, apples, and broccoli. Then, add some nuts, grains, seeds, and beans to make it extra yummy!

Cooking together makes mealtime a very fun and loving time.

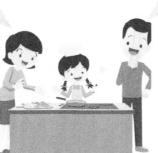

Eating together as a family makes mealtime very special.

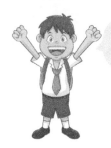
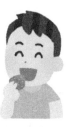

Taste the colors. Feel the brightness!

Color the rainbow of good foods below.

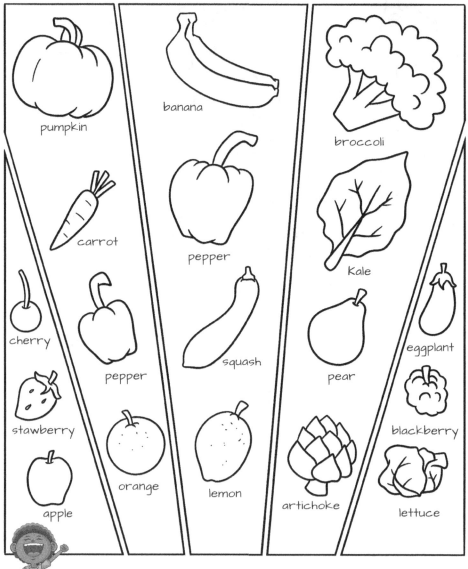

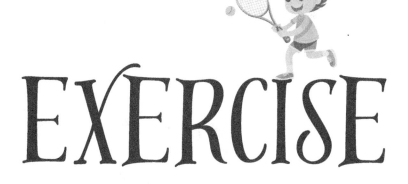

EXERCISE

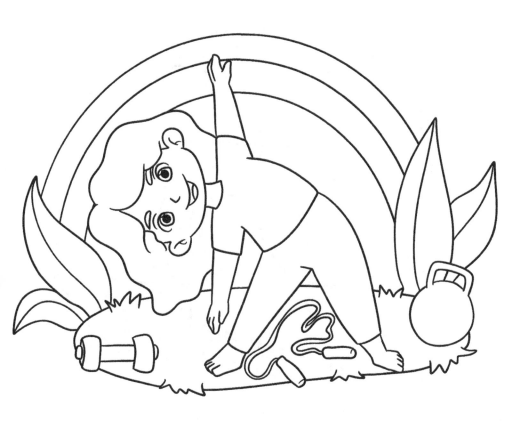

"And Enoch walked with God; and he was not, for God took him."
Genesis 5:24

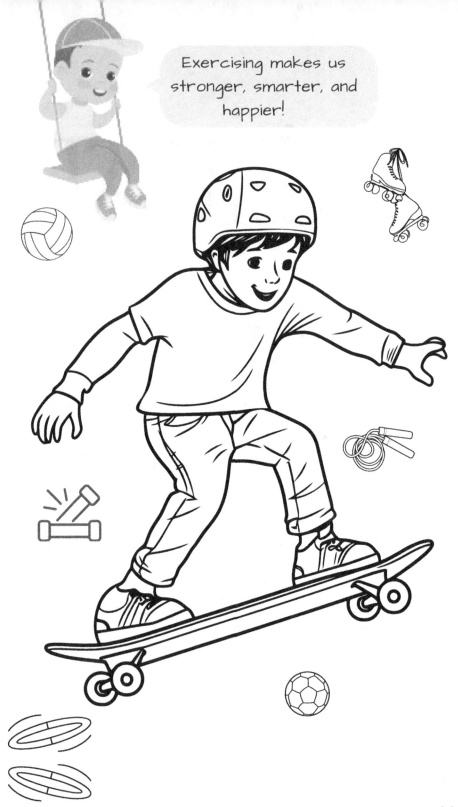

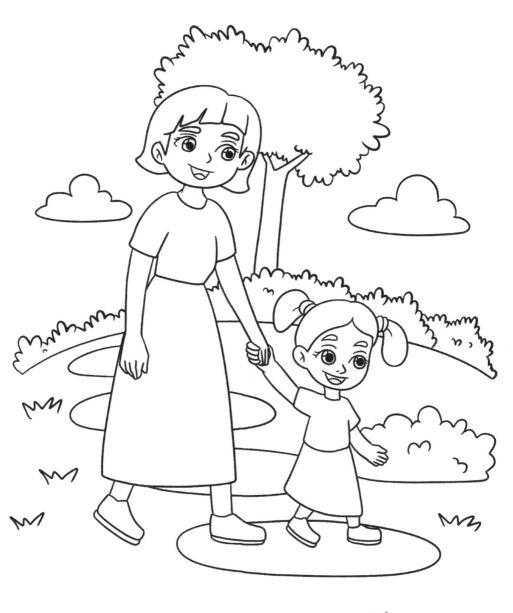

We love walking to school and in nature parks.

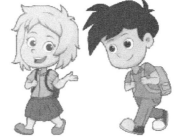

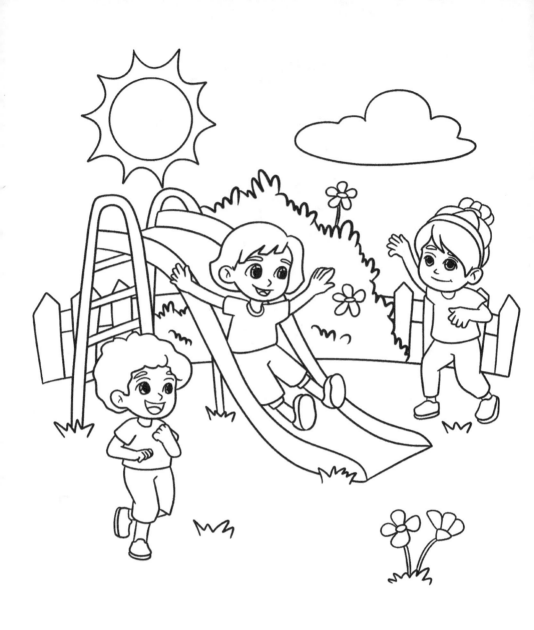

I like exercising at the park. Woohoo!

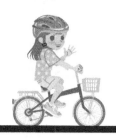

Exercise helps us get better at moving our bodies in different ways and building our confidence.

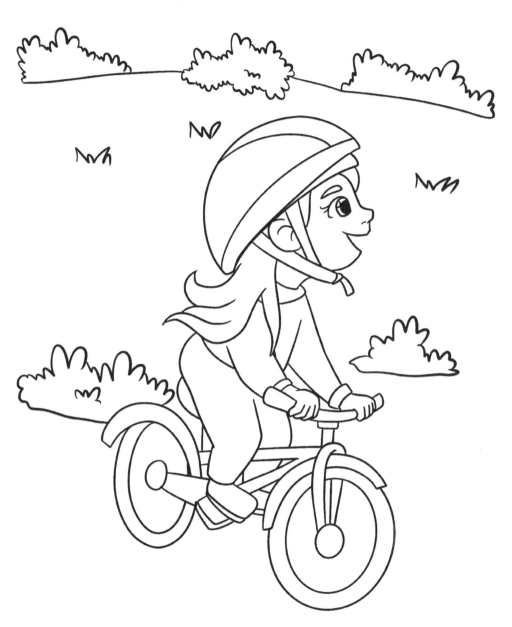

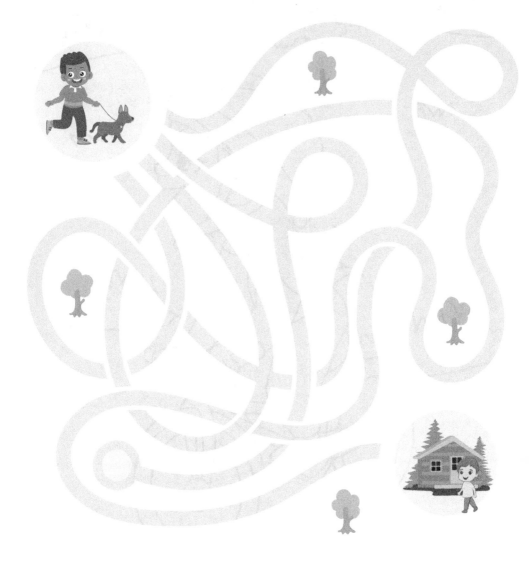

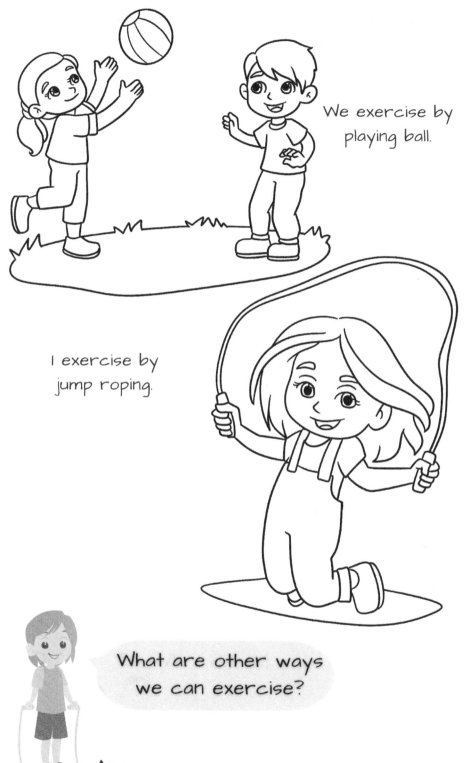

We exercise by playing ball.

I exercise by jump roping.

What are other ways we can exercise?

Ans:_____

Can you find the hidden words showing different ways we can exercise?

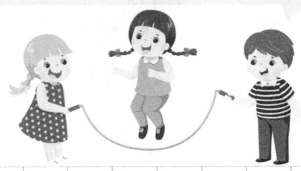

J	F	J	B	M	J	E	Y	K	S
D	D	H	R	I	V	L	R	K	V
F	W	J	U	W	P	N	G	G	L
E	A	U	N	L	K	N	U	E	Y
Y	L	M	N	F	W	I	X	D	P
P	K	P	I	B	Q	J	W	Q	O
L	I	I	N	A	U	B	I	K	E
A	N	N	G	L	H	K	T	B	Y
Y	G	G	S	L	W	F	E	M	C
I	S	C	I	M	S	A	M	B	Q

Ball   Play
Jumping   Running
Bike   Walking

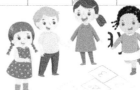

WATER

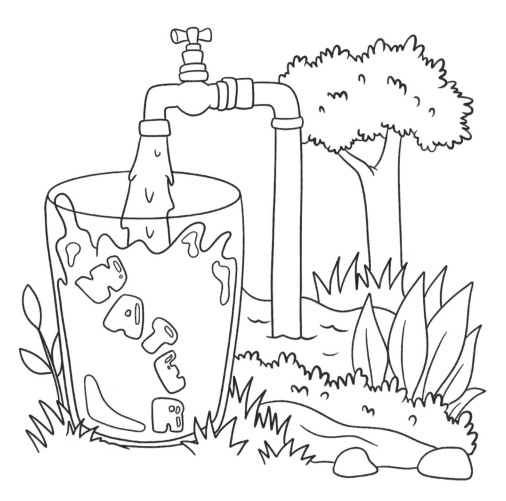

"But whosoever drinks of the water that I shall give him shall never thirst, but the water that I shall give him shall be in him a well of water springing up into everlasting life."
John 4:14

Fun Facts

Did you know that:
Our brain is about 75% water?
90% of our lungs are water?
85% of blood is water?
80% of our skin is water?
75% of muscles are water?
Did you also know that most of our body- about 70%- is made of water?
Interestingly, 70% of the Earth is also water!

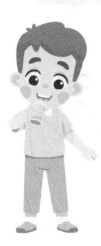

Wow!
We serve a great,
big, wonderful God!

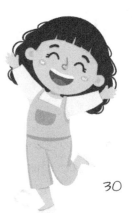

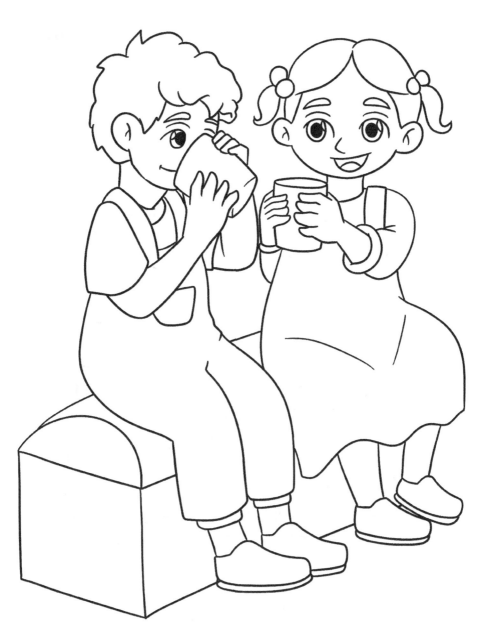

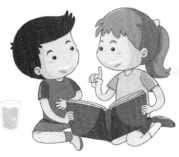

Children under eight years old need at least 4 cups of water every day!

Water:
The clear choice for us.!

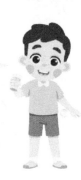

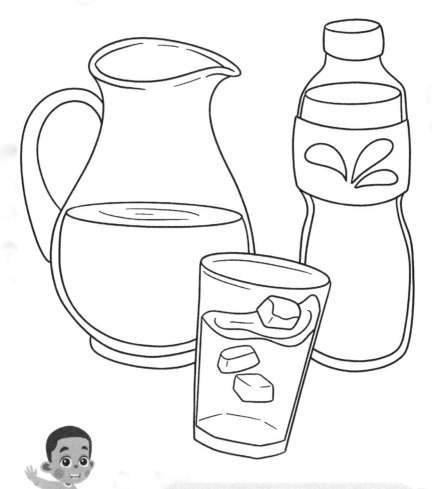

Choose water over soda, energy drinks, sugary drinks, juice, or milk. Your body needs it!

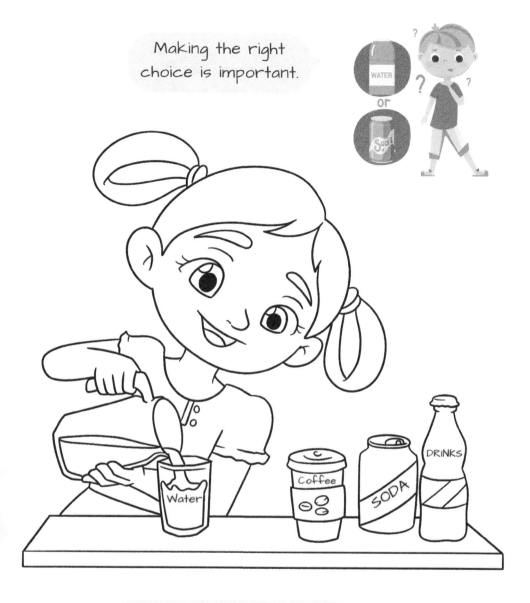

Making the right choice is important.

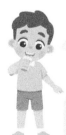
Drinks like soda, coffee, and tea don't give us the water our bodies need.

Drinking water in the morning before breakfast is a healthy practice for everyone.

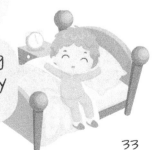

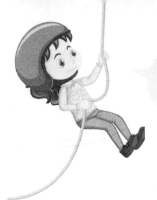

Drinking water gives us energy!

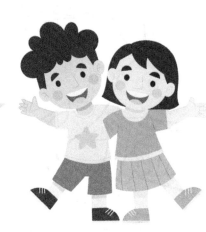

Drinking water makes us happy!

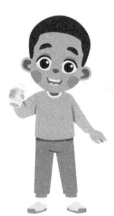

Drinking water prevents headaches and helps our memory!

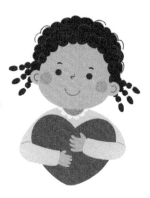

Drinking water keeps us healthy, makes our body feel good, and strengthens our hearts!

SUNLIGHT

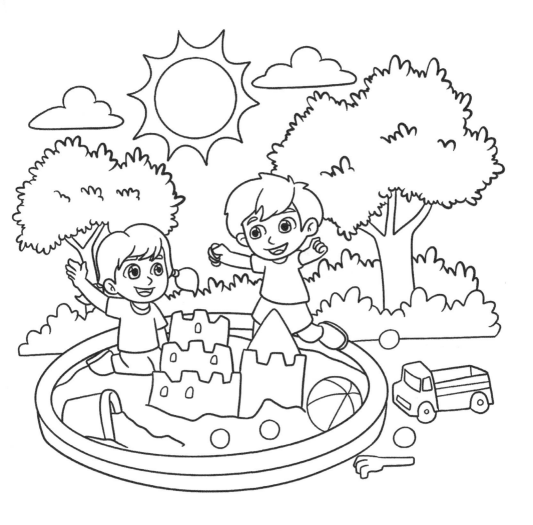

"Truly the light is sweet, and it is pleasant for the eyes to behold the sun"
Ecclesiastes 11:7

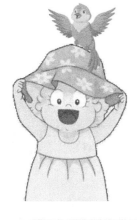

Sunlight gets rid of germs and keeps us healthy.

Sunshine gives us Vitamin D, which makes our bones and teeth strong!

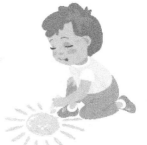
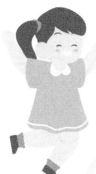

Sunlight improves our mood, helping us to be happy!

Getting daytime sun actually helps you sleep better at night!.

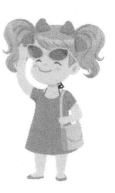
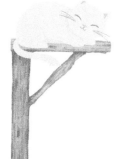

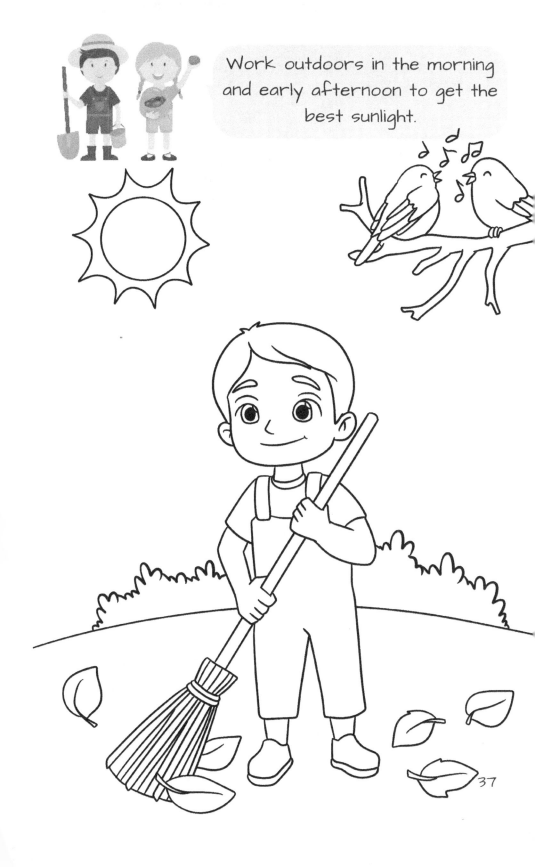

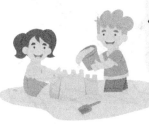

We love going to the beach in the summer, where we get lots of sunlight. But remember to protect your skin from too much direct sun!

We love doing lots of outdoor activities. It makes us happy!

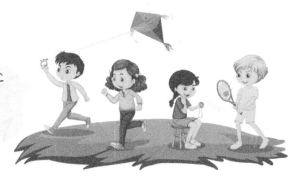

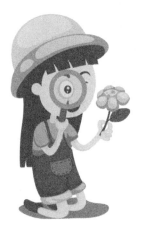

I love exploring the outdoors!

I love to play outdoors with my pet. It is so much fun!

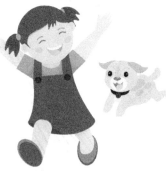

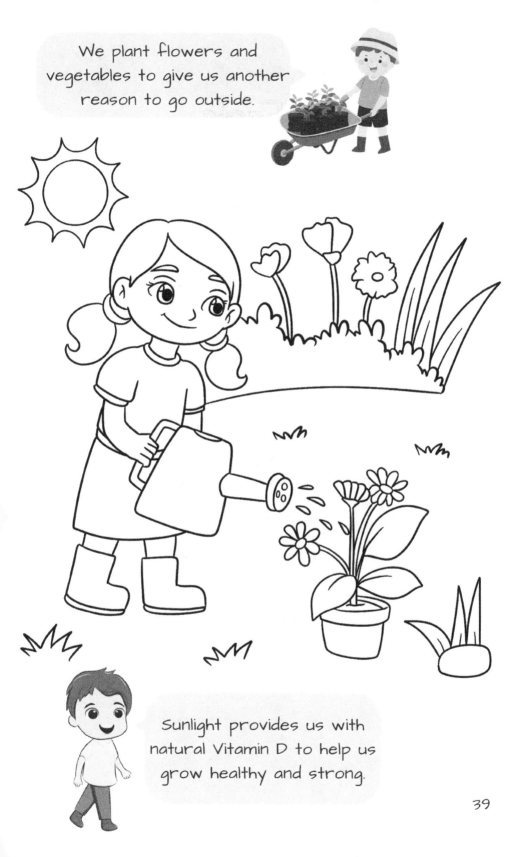

Fun Facts

If it were not for the Sun, there would be no life on the earth. The Sun causes seasons, tides in the oceans, weather, and climates.

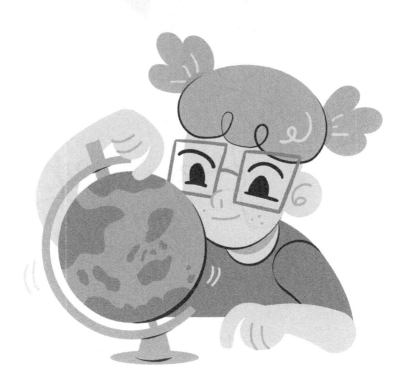

TEMPERANCE

Temperance is self-control.

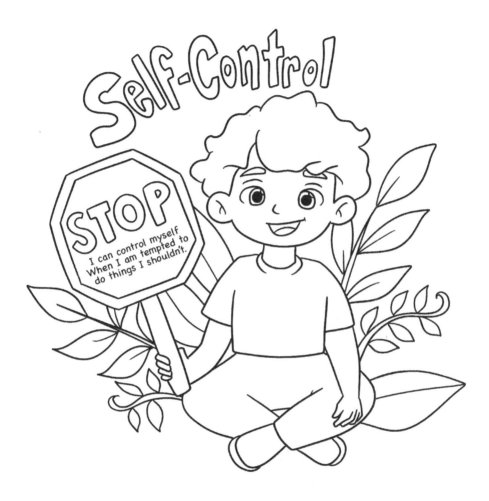

"I beseech you therefore, brethren, by the mercies of God, that ye present your bodies a living sacrifice, holy, acceptable unto God, which is your reasonable service".
Romans 12:1

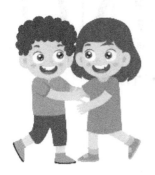

We practice self-control when we can be in charge of our emotions.

The best way to practice self-control is to STOP, THINK, PRAY, and then CHOOSE the right choice.

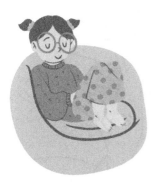

Sometimes, taking a break from activities can help us get better at self-control.

Self-control is knowing you can but deciding you won't!

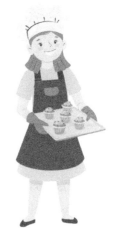

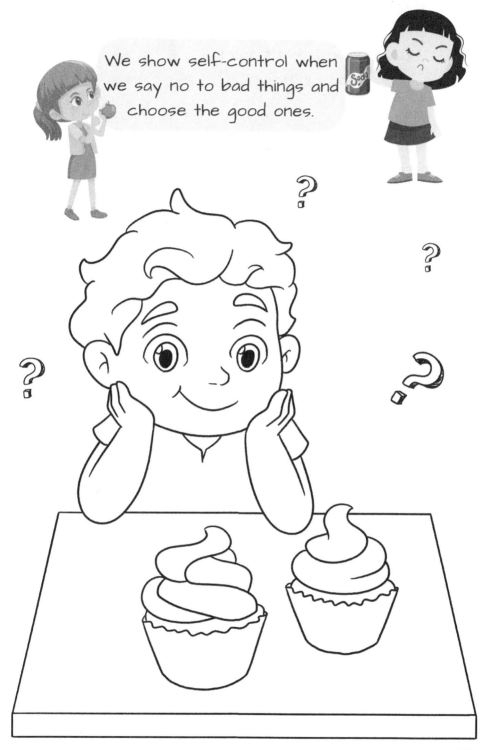

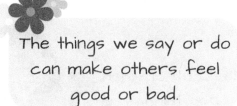
The things we say or do can make others feel good or bad.

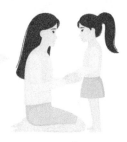

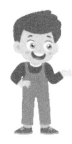
Self-control is also learning what to say and what not to say.

Look at the sentences below. Use a check ✓ or an X to show which ones you should say out loud or which ones you should keep to yourself.

✓ = Say It   X = Don't say it

- [ ] You look nice today.
- [ ] I will share with you.
- [ ] You are so mean!
- [ ] Jesus loves you.
- [ ] It's all your fault.
- [ ] I will help you.
- [ ] You are ugly.
- [ ] May I sit with you?
- [ ] I don't like you.
- [ ] I am better than you.
- [ ] I would love to play with you.
- [ ] I will never talk to you, ever.

Self-control

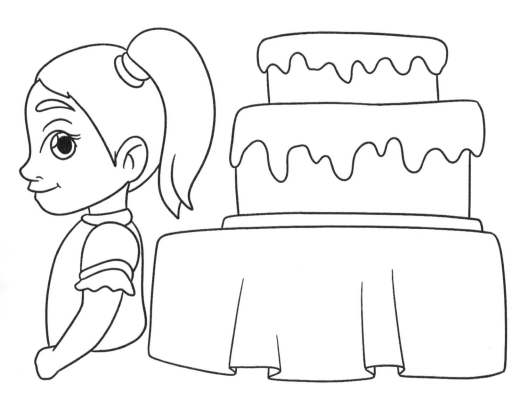

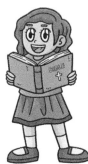

The more we get to know Jesus, the more self-control we have.

Fill in the blanks to spell out the guide to self-control

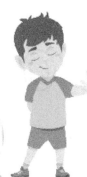

S _ O _

TH _ N _

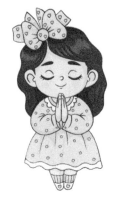

P _ _ _

CH _ _ S _

Answer clue on page 42

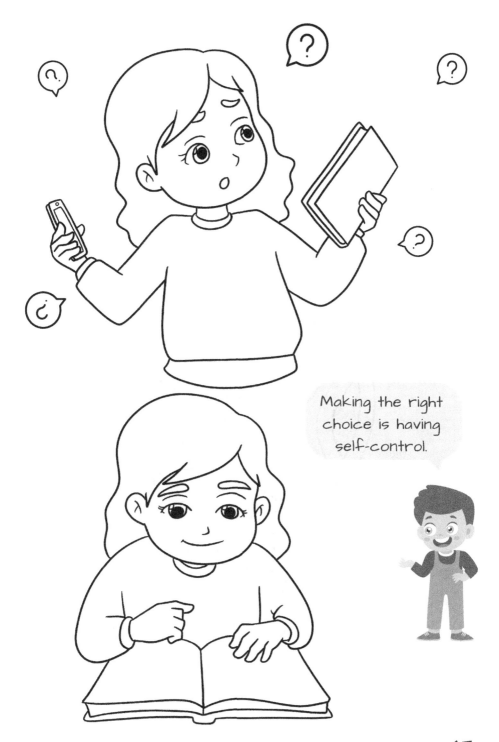

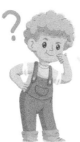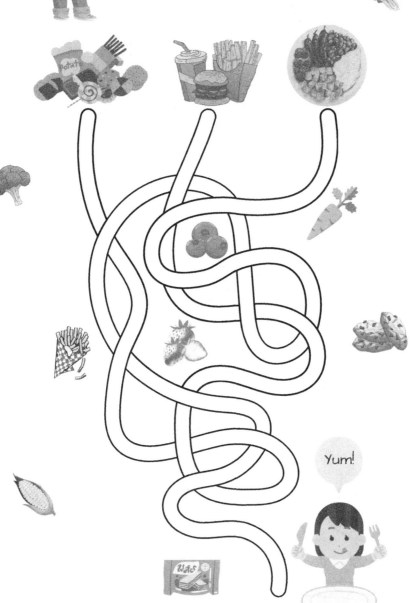

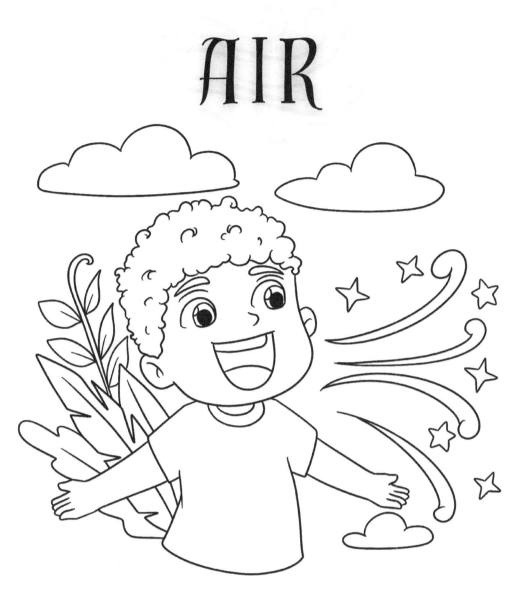

AIR

"And the LORD God formed man of the dust of the ground, and breathed into his nostrils the breath of life; and man became a living soul."
Genesis 2:7

Why is fresh air so good for us?

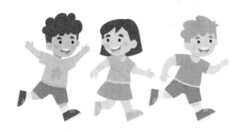

Fresh air makes us happier.

Fresh air cleans our lungs.

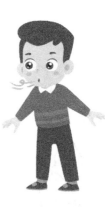

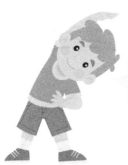

Fresh air makes our immune system strong, helping us not get sick.

Fresh air gives us more energy and helps us to focus better.

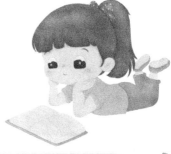

Fresh air helps us sleep better at night.

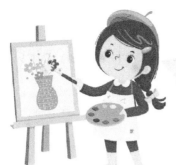

Fresh air helps us to be calm, relaxed, and happy!

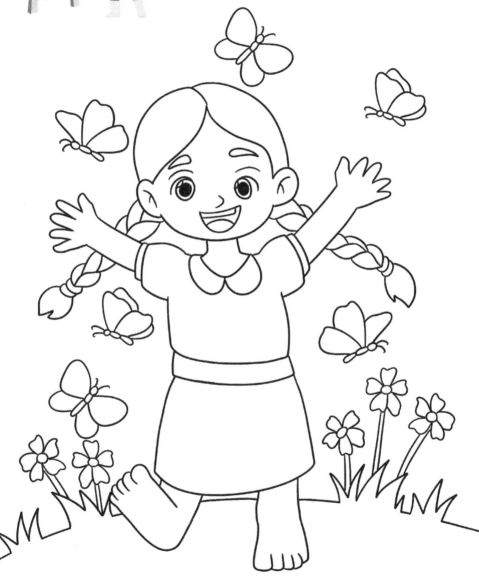

Take a deep breath; it's free!

What are some ways we can get fresh air?

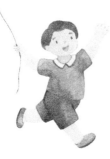

We get fresh air by doing activities outdoors, like playing, exercising, walking, hiking, and camping.

We get fresh air by opening our windows.

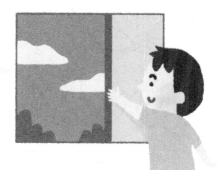

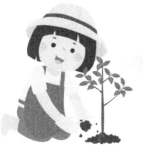

We get fresh air by planting flowers and trees and having certain plants in our house, like peace lilies and spider plants, which help clean the air.

We get fresh air when we take deep breaths in places with good airflow.

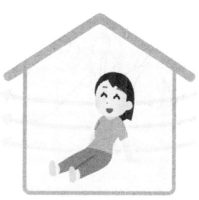

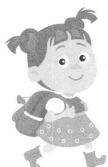

I like hiking in nature parks with my parents, where the air is fresh and clean.

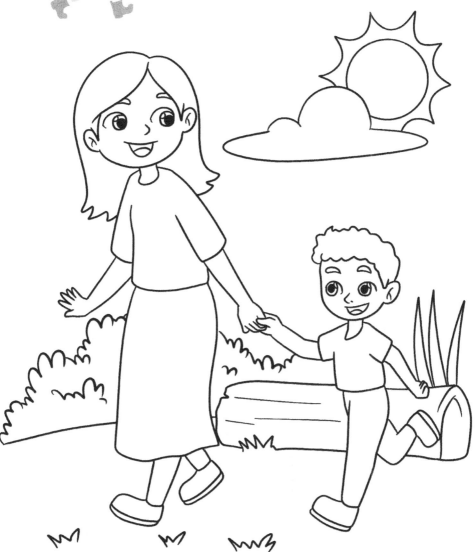

Some air can be dangerous to our bodies!

Air pollution is when the air we breathe gets dirty with things like gases or chemicals.

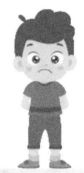

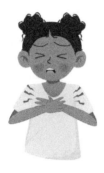

Stay away from dirty air like smoke, chemicals, gas smells, strong fumes, mold, and stinky garbage.

Here is a simple deep breathing exercise to help to relax your mind and body:

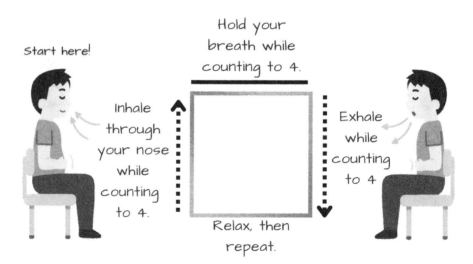

Start here!

Inhale through your nose while counting to 4.

Hold your breath while counting to 4.

Exhale while counting to 4

Relax, then repeat.

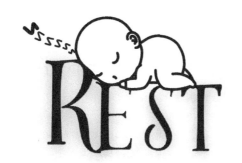

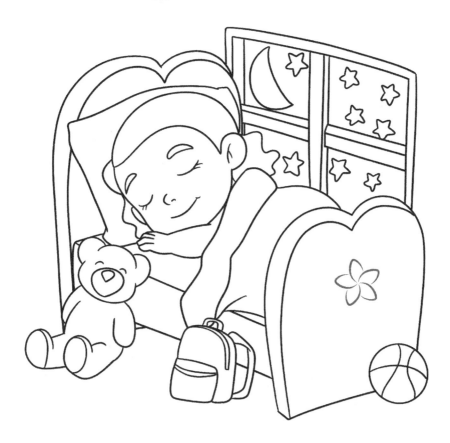

"Come unto me, all ye that labour and are heavy laden, and I will give you rest. Take my yoke upon you, and learn of me; for I am meek and lowly in heart: and ye shall find rest unto your souls. For My yoke is easy, and My burden is light".
Matthew 11:28-30

Why do we need proper rest?

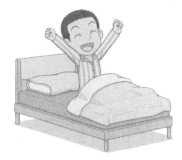

Proper rest helps us to be better-behaved and less anxious.

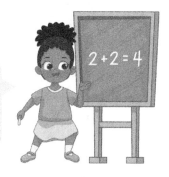

Getting enough sleep helps us feel happier, remember things better, stay focused, pay attention, and learn new things easier.

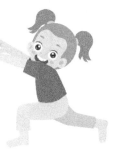

Proper rest helps our bodies stay strong and healthy, making us less likely to get sick.

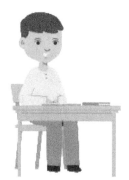

Proper rest helps our brains work well so we can remember what we learn.

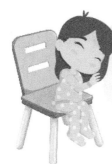

Our mind and body need rest to recharge, repair, and stay healthy.

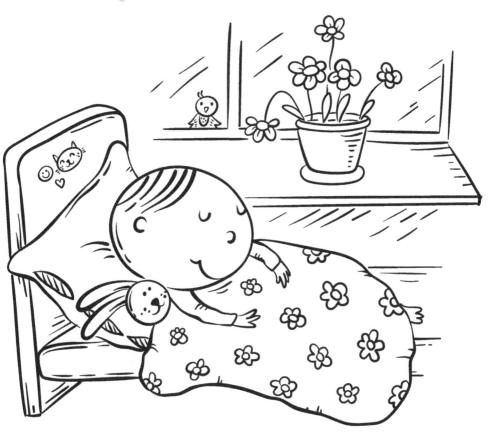

Here are some ways to get better rest naturally.

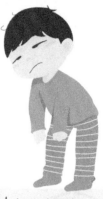

Good sleeping habits help us get a better night's sleep.

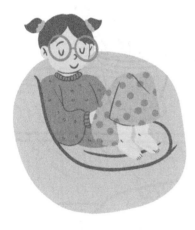

Schedule playtime outdoors with breaks for rest and quiet time.

Make sure you give your brain time to rest and calm down before bedtime.

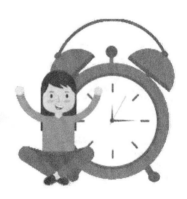

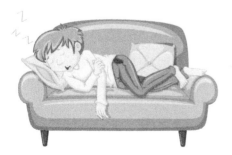

Taking a nap during the day helps us to be in a better mood.

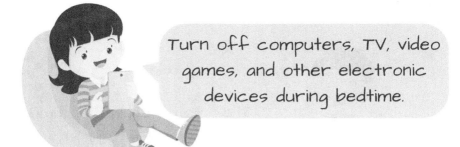

Turn off computers, TV, video games, and other electronic devices during bedtime.

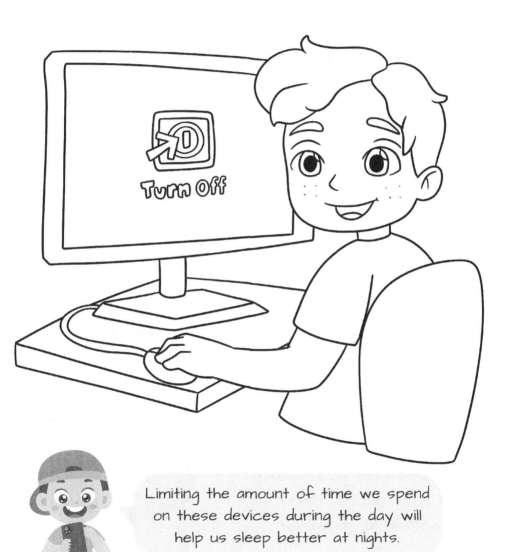

Limiting the amount of time we spend on these devices during the day will help us sleep better at nights.

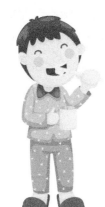

Stick to a regular bedtime routine every night.

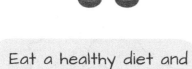 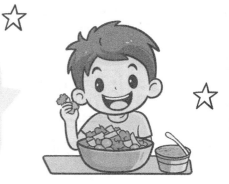

Eat a healthy diet and don't have big meals, caffeine, or sugary treats before bedtime.

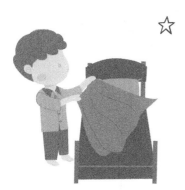

Don't eat too late or close to bedtime.

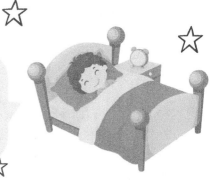

Getting proper rest at night helps us feel wide awake and focused at school so we can learn better!

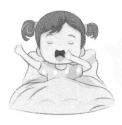

Can you find all the words hidden in the puzzle below?

LET YOUR SLEEP BE SWEET

s	m	n	h	a	b	i	t	h	c
n	a	p	t	i	m	e	j	e	l
z	o	r	e	s	t	i	k	a	u
n	o	q	z	f	i	s	m	l	x
r	w	q	o	j	h	e	b	t	t
m	b	e	d	t	i	m	e	h	x
c	x	g	s	l	e	e	p	y	a
j	g	q	i	l	e	a	r	n	m
g	g	p	v	n	j	e	x	e	p
l	a	n	i	g	h	t	l	j	o

bedtime
learn
habit
healthy

naptime
night
rest
sleep

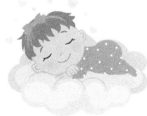

Fun Facts

Did you know that children need about 10 hours of sleep every night? Proper sleep helps us behave better, learn better, and have healthier brains, bodies, and minds.

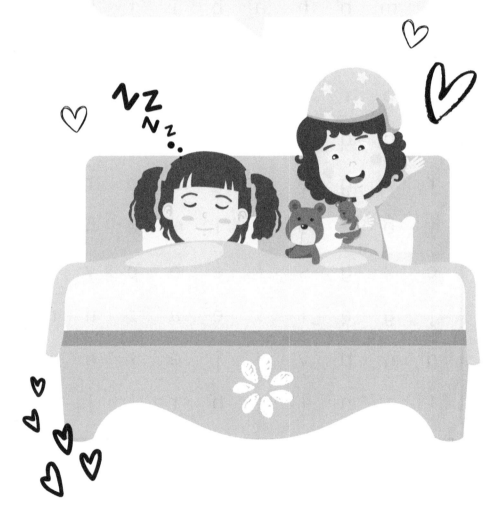

TRUST IN GOD

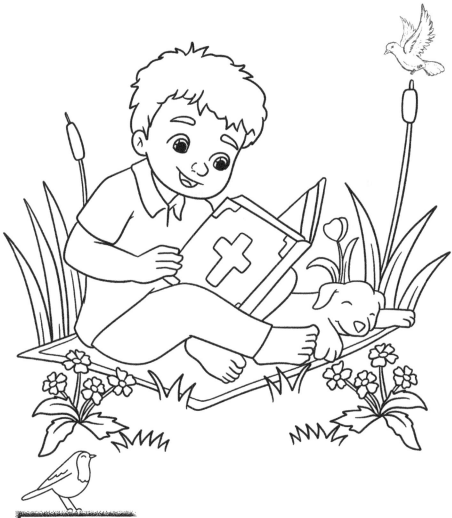

"Trust in the Lord with all your heart and lean not on your own understanding. In all your ways, acknowledge Him, and He will direct our path".
Proverbs 3:5-6

God helps us make right choices.

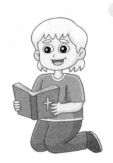

The Bible has amazing stories about God helping His people feel brave and strong so they can make good choices!

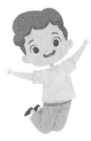

Jesus knows what will make us happy, healthy, and strong. He will give us the strength to follow what's right.

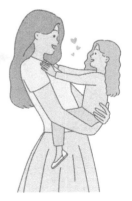

If we make a mistake, Jesus will forgive us when we ask Him. He helps us stop doing bad things and start doing good things instead!

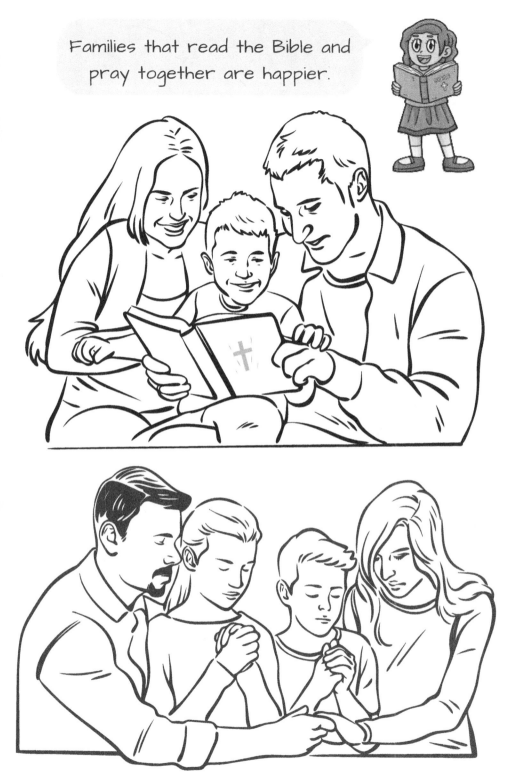

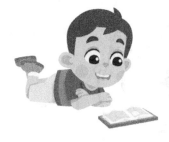

The Bible is God's love letter to us, filled with beautiful promises that makes us feel happy, safe, and encouraged.

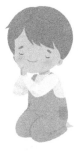

Pray and read the Bible and let someone know how wonderful God is.

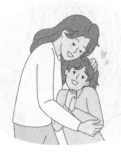

God loves us so much that He created this beautiful world and provided us with the things of nature for our health, healing, and happiness.

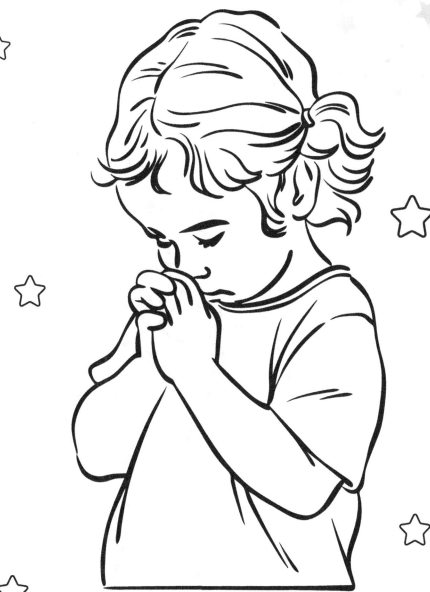

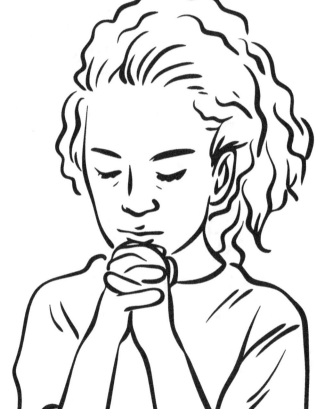

Heavenly Father, thank you for helping me stay healthy and strong. Help me follow these 8 steps to be happier and healthier and help me share them with others.
In Jesus' name, Amen!

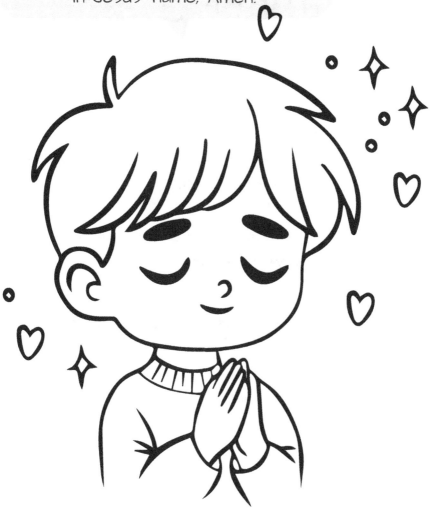

"Beloved, I wish above all things that you may prosper and be in health, even as your soul prosper."
3 John 2

Thank you

Your order made our day! We hope we make yours.

We are thrilled to share this experience with you, and we hope that your child will find it enjoyable. Please do not hesitate to explore more books from our collection.

If you have any questions, contact us anytime. We'd love to hear from you.

purebluepublications@gmail.com

Made in the USA
Middletown, DE
10 August 2024